TONSIL STONES

UNDERSTANDING TONSIL STONES

PERFECTLY

DR. J. WALLER

Contents

INTRODUCTION

The two little lumps of tissue at the back of the throat, the tonsils, can develop tiny, white or yellowish calcifications called tonsil stones, or tonsilloliths. Debris, dead cells, mucus, and germs that build up in the tonsils' crypts or pockets usually make up these stones.

Important details regarding tonsils include:

Formation: Debris that becomes lodged in the tonsil crypts, such as food particles, dead cells, and bacteria, leads to the development of tonsil stones. These substances solidify and calcify over time to produce tiny, frequently odorous stones.

Symptoms: Although symptoms of tonsil stones may not always be apparent, common indications include painful throats, trouble swallowing, bad breath (halitosis), and a feeling that something is lodged in the throat.

Risk factors: Those who have a history of recurrent tonsillitis or who have larger tonsils are at a higher risk of acquiring tonsil stones. Chronic sinus problems and poor dental hygiene might also be factors.

Diagnosis: A physical examination of the tonsils and throat is typically used to identify tonsil stones. To determine the size of the stones, imaging studies like CT scans may occasionally be carried out.

Options for Treatment:

At-Home Remedies: Using an oral irrigator, gargling frequently, and maintaining proper hydration can all help to prevent or dislodge small tonsil stones.

Manual Removal: A medical practitioner may use specialized instruments to manually remove larger tonsil stones.

Tonsillectomy: A tonsillectomy, or the surgical removal of the tonsils, may be considered in situations that are severe or recurrent.

Prevention: To lessen the chance of tonsil stones forming, maintain proper oral hygiene, drink plenty of water, and abstain from tobacco products.

Even while tonsil stones are usually benign, their accompanying symptoms and aesthetic problems can make them irritating. It's critical for people dealing with tonsil stone problems to comprehend how they originate, what symptoms they cause, and what treatments are available.

CHAPTER ONE

Origins and Development

Many compounds build up and calcify in the tonsil crypts, resulting in tonsil stones, also known as tonsilloliths. There are multiple contributing elements that contribute to the multifactorial cause of tonsil stone production.

Accumulation of Debris:

On their surface, tonsils have tiny crypts or pockets. Over time, detritus such as germs, mucus, dead cells, and food particles can gather in these crypts.

Activity of Bacteria:

The immune system's tonsils are home to lymphocytes that aid in the defense against infections. The material that is trapped in the tonsil crypts can interact with bacteria, including those that are naturally found in the mouth. The calcification of the debris and the development of biofilms may result from this interaction.

Bad Dental Hygiene

Poor dental hygiene habits, such as sporadic flossing and brushing, might promote the growth of oral germs. Debris accumulation in tonsil crypts can be attributed to inadequate dental hygiene practices.

Prolonged Tonsillitis:

Tonsil stones may occur more frequently in people with a history of recurrent tonsillitis. Debris can accumulate and calcify in an environment that is facilitated by chronic tonsil irritation.

Huge Crypts of Tonsils:

Individual tonsil crypts differ in size and structure. People who have larger tonsil crypts might be more prone to debris buildup, which could create an environment that is favorable for the production of tonsil stones.

Parched Mouth:

The accumulation of bacteria and debris in the mouth may be facilitated by decreased salivary flow or dry mouth, which may raise the risk of tonsil stones developing.

Nutritional Elements:

Tonsil stones may be caused by certain dietary factors, such as a diet heavy in dairy products or low in meals high in water. These ingredients may cause the creation of thicker mucus.

Molecular Predisposition:

A person's vulnerability to tonsil stones may be influenced by their genetic makeup. Genetic factors may make certain people more susceptible to tonsil stones.

A number of these variables combine to generate tonsil stones, which frequently develop gradually. Even though they are usually not harmful, they can still result in discomfort and unpleasant symptoms like bad breath. Tonsil stones can be prevented and treated by controlling contributory factors, maintaining proper oral hygiene, and getting medical care when necessary.

Not everyone experiences symptoms associated with tonsil stones, or tonsilloliths, and some people may be unaware that they have them. When symptoms do appear, though, they may include:

Halitosis, or bad breath:

Persistent foul breath is one of the most typical signs of tonsil stones. The stones smell bad because they are home to bacteria and dirt.

Throat Pain:

A sore throat can result from tonsil stones irritating and inflaming the tonsils. This symptom could be most apparent after swallowing.

Having Trouble Swallowing:

A sensation of difficulty or discomfort during swallowing may be brought on by larger tonsil stones or a buildup of smaller stones.

Evident kidney stones:

There are instances where people may feel or see the tonsil stones on the tonsil surface. The stones can seem as hard, tiny lumps and are frequently white or yellowish in appearance.

Pain in the Ears:

Sometimes, transferred pain from tonsil stones might induce discomfort in the ears. The tonsils and ears share neural pathways, which could be the cause of this.

Coughing

If the tonsil stones irritate the throat or set off the gag reflex, persistent coughing may result.

Taste of Metal:

A metallic or disagreeable taste in the mouth is reported by some tonsil stone sufferers, and this can be linked to the stones themselves.

Inflamed Tonsils:

The sense of something caught in the throat may be exacerbated by swollen tonsils caused by the buildup of debris and inflammation.

Debris White on Tonsils:

People may observe white or yellowish debris on the tonsil surface in addition to obvious tonsil stones.

It's crucial to remember that not everyone with tonsil stones has symptoms, and that symptoms might differ in intensity. While some tonsil stones are tiny and go unnoticed, others could cause more noticeable symptoms. People should seek medical attention if they have ongoing symptoms or discomfort in order to receive an accurate diagnosis and the best course of treatment.

Preventive Techniques

Although totally preventing tonsil stones isn't always feasible, there are several tactics that can lessen the likelihood of them forming as well as the discomfort they cause. Here are a few precautions to take:

Maintaining Good Dental Hygiene

Keep up a strict oral hygiene regimen that includes using an antiseptic mouthwash, flossing, and frequent brushing of your teeth and tongue. This lessens the amount of germs that accumulates in the mouth.

Gargling

Periodically gargle with saltwater or a non-alcoholic mouthwash. Gargling can lessen the chance of tonsil stone formation by helping to remove dirt and bacteria from the tonsil crypts.

Maintain Hydration:

To ensure sufficient salivation throughout the day, sip water frequently. Saliva aids in mouth cleaning and keeps particles from building up.

Steer clear of tobacco products:

Smoking increases the chance of tonsil stones and might aggravate dry mouth. For dental health, giving up tobacco use or avoiding its products can be advantageous.

Modifications to Diet:

Eat a nutritious, well-balanced diet rich in a range of fruits, vegetables, and whole grains. Steer clear of dairy items in excess since this can increase mucus production.

Frequent dental examinations:

Make an appointment for routine dental examinations to keep an eye on your oral health and catch any problems early. Dental professionals can offer advice on good oral hygiene procedures.

Employ a Flosser:

Oral irrigators and water flossers are useful tools for clearing debris and cleansing the tonsil crypts. Include these in your daily dental hygiene regimen.

Don't Drink Too Much Alcohol:

Drinking too much alcohol can cause dehydration, which raises the possibility of tonsil stones developing. Restrict alcohol consumption while staying hydrated.

Reduce or Give Up Smoking:

If you smoke, think about cutting back on your tobacco use. Smoking raises the risk of bacterial development in the mouth and can aggravate dry mouth.

Methods for Removing Tonsil Stones:

Regular removal methods, like gently pushing on the tonsils with a cotton swab, may help avoid the buildup of material in those who are prone to tonsil stones.

It is noteworthy that people should seek medical guidance for additional evaluation and proper care if they have recurrent tonsil stone irritation or chronic symptoms. A medical expert may suggest more focused treatments in certain situations or, in more serious ones, a tonsillectomy (the surgical removal of the tonsils).

CHAPTER TWO

Fixes and Upkeep at Home

Tonsil stones can be managed and the symptoms they cause can be lessened with a few simple home cures and upkeep techniques. These treatments can be useful in avoiding tonsil stones from forming and reducing discomfort, even though they might not completely remove them. Here are some maintenance guidelines and at-home cures:

Frequently Gargling:

Gargling with saltwater or using a mouthwash without alcohol can aid in clearing the tonsil crypts of debris, germs, and tonsil stones. You can perform this routinely as part of your dental hygiene.

Maintain Hydration:

To ensure sufficient salivation throughout the day, sip water frequently. Staying hydrated helps avoid dry mouth, which can lead to the development of tonsil stones.

Oral Hydration:

To gently clean the tonsil crypts, use an oral irrigator or water flosser. This may work well to remove debris and stop the buildup of substances that cause tonsil stones.

Light Tonsil Massage:

To remove any apparent tonsil stones, gently massage the tonsils with a cotton swab or your toothbrush. Take care not to irritate or hurt anyone.

Optimal Dental Hygiene Procedures:

Keep up a strict and consistent oral hygiene regimen that includes cleaning your tongue, teeth, and roof of your mouth. Flossing aids in the removal of debris in between teeth.

Steer clear of irritants:

Strong mouthwashes with alcohol and other irritants should be avoided or minimized since they can exacerbate dry mouth. Instead, use mouthwashes without alcohol.

Scraping of the tongue:

To clean the tongue's surface of debris and microorganisms, use a tongue scraper. This promotes general dental hygiene.

Probiotics:

Think about taking probiotic supplements or including foods high in probiotics in your diet. Probiotics might assist in keeping the proper ratio of bacteria in the mouth.

Modifications to Diet:

A balanced diet that includes a range of whole grains, fruits, and vegetables is recommended. If you observe a connection between dairy consumption and the development of tonsil stones, reduce your intake of dairy products.

Add Humidity to the Air:

To add moisture to the air in your bedroom, use a humidifier. This can lessen the chance of developing tonsil stones and prevent dry mouth.

Give Up Smoking:

If you smoke, think about cutting back on your tobacco use. Smoking raises the risk of bacterial development in the mouth and can aggravate dry mouth.

It's crucial to remember that the goals of these natural treatments are to control symptoms and lower the likelihood of tonsil stones developing. For additional assessment and suitable treatment, people should consult a doctor if they have extreme discomfort, repeated tonsil stones, or ongoing symptoms. A medical expert might suggest a tonsillectomy or more focused treatments in specific situations.

When people have prolonged symptoms or discomfort and preventive measures are ineffective, medical procedures for tonsil stones may be advised. Various interventions, such as the following, may be recommended by healthcare professionals based on the frequency and severity of tonsil stones:

Removal by Hand by a Medical Expert:

When tonsil stones are visible and easily removed, a medical professional such as an ENT specialist may use specialized instruments to manually remove the stones.

Curette or Irrigation with Water:

To remove and remove tonsil stones, a medical expert may use a curette or water irrigation. Usually, this process is carried out in a clinical environment.

Cryptolysis of Laser Tonsils:

The process known as "laser cryptolysis" involves using a laser to shallow the tonsil crypts and smooth the tonsil surface. By doing this, the buildup of stones and debris may be avoided.

Tonsillectomy:

In extreme situations or when recurring tonsil stones are causing a great deal of discomfort, a tonsillectomy could be advised. A tonsillectomy, which involves surgically removing the tonsils, is seen to be a more long-term fix.

Tonsillectomy by comblation:

Coblation tonsillectomy is a surgical method in which the tonsils are removed using radiofrequency energy. In comparison to more conventional tonsillectomy techniques, it seeks to lessen postoperative pain.

Antibiotics:

A medical professional may recommend medications to treat the infection and lessen inflammation if tonsil stones are linked to an underlying infection, such as tonsillitis.

It's crucial to remember that, even while medical procedures can be successful, they are usually saved for situations in which tonsil stones result in serious symptoms or consequences. The individual's general health, the intensity of symptoms, and the frequency of tonsil stone recurrence all play a role in the decision to pursue a specific strategy.

Those who are uncomfortable or have ongoing tonsil stone symptoms should speak with a medical practitioner for a comprehensive assessment and tailored advice. Getting expert counsel guarantees that the intervention selected is suitable for the particular situation and yields the best results.

Taking Care of the Basis Conditions

Preventing the recurrence of tonsil stones requires addressing the underlying problems that contribute to their creation. In order to address any potential underlying causes, take into account the following:

How to Treat Tonsillitis:

Antibiotics to treat bacterial infections may be a suitable treatment if tonsillitis recurs often. If tonsillitis is severe or chronic, further testing and even a tonsillectomy are necessary.

Handling Allergies:

Allergies may raise the risk of tonsil stone formation by causing nasal congestion and postnasal drip. Using nasal sprays, allergy immunotherapy, or antihistamines to treat allergies can be helpful.

Treatment for Gastroesophageal Reflux Disease (GERD):

Stomach acid can reflux into the throat as a result of GERD, irritating it and perhaps creating tonsil stones. It may be advised to make dietary adjustments, lifestyle adjustments, and drug changes to control GERD symptoms.

Drinking plenty of water

Since dehydration can exacerbate tonsil stones, it's critical to maintain adequate hydrated to avoid dry mouth. Water should be consumed in moderation throughout the day.

Practices for Oral Hygiene:

Stress the importance of maintaining proper oral hygiene, which includes flossing and routinely cleaning your teeth, tongue, and roof of your mouth. Bacteria in the mouth can be decreased by using an antiseptic mouthwash.

Modifications to Diet:

It might be beneficial to change the diet to incorporate more whole grains, fruits, and vegetables while reducing dairy products. Some people discover that dietary modifications affect their production of mucus.

Probiotics:

Including foods or supplements high in probiotics may help keep the bacteria in your mouth in a healthy balance and lower your chance of getting sick.

Give Up Smoking:

Smoking raises the possibility of oral bacterial growth and can aggravate dry mouth. Reducing or giving up tobacco use is good for your dental health in general.

Management of Prolonged Sinus Problems:

Prolonged sinus problems may cause postnasal drip, which can act as a source of material for the development of tonsils. It could be essential to treat sinus problems with medicine or other measures.

Collaborating closely with medical professionals is crucial in order to detect and treat any underlying issues that may be causing tonsil stones. The best course of action for treating underlying causes and preventing recurrent tonsil stones can be determined with the aid of a thorough evaluation that includes a complete medical history and examination.

CHAPTER THREE

Handling Embarrassment

Tonsil stones can be embarrassing, particularly if they result in symptoms that are obvious, including foul breath or evident debris on the tonsils. The following coping mechanisms will help you deal with the shame that comes with tonsil stones:

Recall that you are not alone:

Tonsil stones are rather frequent and affect a lot of people at some point. It can be comforting to know that you're not the only one struggling with this problem.

Honest Communication

If it makes you feel better, think about talking to close friends or family about the problem. Fostering a supportive environment and reducing emotions of humiliation can both be achieved through open communication.

Consult a Professional:

To address the underlying causes of tonsil stones, consult with a medical practitioner, such as an ENT specialist. They are able to offer managerial advice and suggestions for possible actions.

Sustain Proper Dental Hygiene:

Stress the need of maintaining proper dental hygiene to reduce the effects of tonsil stones. Using an antiseptic mouthwash, brushing, and flossing on a regular basis will help lessen symptoms.

Apply Mouth Fresheners:

Stock up on sugar-free mints or breath fresheners to help with tonsil stone-related foul breath. This can offer a prompt resolution when required.

Maintain Hydration:

By sustaining enough saliva production, drinking lots of water lowers the risk of tonsil stones and dry mouth.

Exercise Prudence:

Use caution in social circumstances if you're worried about noticeable tonsil stones. Steer clear of bringing up the matter, and if necessary, excuse yourself quietly for a short while.

Use Products for Breath Freshening:

To treat foul breath brought on by tonsil stones, try breath freshening items like sugar-free gum or breath sprays.

Bring a Bottle of Water:

If you feel the urge to freshen your breath, carrying a water bottle with you lets you stay hydrated.

Learn for Yourself:

Gaining knowledge about tonsil stones, their causes, and the many therapeutic options will enable you to confidently confront the problem.

Think About Hiring a Professional:

If your self-esteem or quality of life are greatly affected by tonsil stones, you might want to contact a therapist or counselor for professional assistance. They can offer you support and direction.

Keep in mind that everyone experiences difficulties or embarrassment related to some aspects of their health. Being proactive in managing tonsil stones and getting help when required can help one feel in charge and self-assured. If embarrassment starts to interfere with your life or gets too much, go to a mental health or medical professional who can provide help and assistance.

CONCLUSION

In conclusion, tonsil stones are a frequent and usually innocuous condition, despite the fact that they can be embarrassing. The symptoms of bad breath, sore throat, and a sensation of something trapped in the throat can be caused by these tiny, calcified deposits in the tonsil crypts.

Tonsil stone management is a mix of lifestyle modifications, over-the-counter medications, and, occasionally, surgical procedures. Tonsil stone formation can be avoided by practicing good oral hygiene, drinking plenty of water, and treating underlying conditions like allergies or chronic tonsillitis.

If social settings or obvious symptoms cause you to feel embarrassed, keep in mind that getting support from trusted people in your life as well as medical specialists can help you cope with the issue better. Dealing with this disease requires open communication, tonsil stone education, and a proactive attitude to oral health.

If your quality of life is being negatively impacted by tonsil stones or if they are causing chronic discomfort, you should definitely seek the advice of a healthcare provider for a comprehensive assessment. Tonsil stones can be successfully navigated and managed by people with the correct knowledge and assistance, enhancing their overall oral health and well-being.

THE END